Reboot

Reboot

Lessons Learned On My ACL Journey

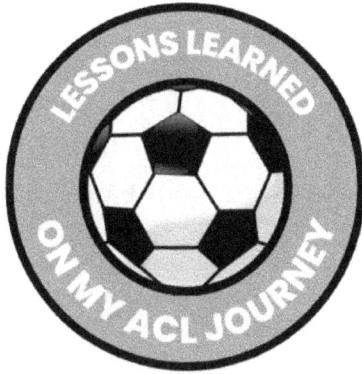

Avigail Morris

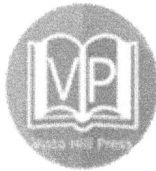

Vista Hill Press

A Division of Five Minute Network, LLC

Los Angeles

REBOOT:
Lessons Learned On My ACL Journey

Copyright © 2023 by Avigail Morris

Published by
Vista Hill Press
A Division of Five Minute Network, LLC
907 Westwood Blvd., Suite 405
Los Angeles, CA 90024

First Edition: 2023
Logo design: Avigail Morris
Cover design: Bojan Rekovic
Book design: Julia Bleck
Library of Congress Cataloging-in-Publication Data is available.
ISBN-13: 978-0-9968377-6-7
ISBN-13: 978-0-9968377-7-4

For Mom and Dad—for encouraging me to never give up
and always follow my dreams wherever they take me.

~

For Camp Kesem—for being my home away from home.

~

For all the teenage athletes on their journeys.

CONTENTS

INTRODUCTION

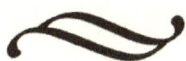

D ear Friend:

Pop. That word was just a word until the very moment when the sound echoed through every cell of my being. I had many friends who've heard the sound and told me about it. The terror. The heartbreak. The feeling of loss. The grief. Some of us were fortunate and never heard that sound and I had always wished that I would be so lucky. However, that's not how life works. Sometimes I wish life would be so easy. Having everything go my way. All the balls go into the net. All the games go our way. Forrest Gump once said that life is like a box of chocolates, and you don't know what you're going to get each time. That thought raced through my mind right as the echo of the pop started to wane. That thought was followed by fear. The fear that my life was about to change. Who was I? I was that star soccer player. I was the kid who scored 12 goals in a game back in the day. Well, I knew things were about to change. I didn't need an MRI or a doctor to tell me. All I needed to hear was that sound. That sound of everything breaking up; tearing apart. The core of who I had been was being torn up and in that moment, all I could think about was "things would never be the same again." This is my story, my journey.

I know that my story isn't unique. There are so many teenagers out there just like me. Like me, they thought they knew exactly who they were. The star athlete. The star musician. The star whatever. And in a single moment, everything changed. This book is my story, my journey, but maybe it's yours too. In a sense, we're all on the same journey; from the sound of that pop to finding out who we really are. Let me start from the beginning ...

Avigail

My ACL Journey Begins:
When Everything Changes

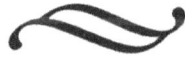

I am never going to play soccer again. That is the first thing that crosses my mind as I feel and hear a pop in my left knee. There is about 15 minutes left of practice on Wednesday, March 30, 2022. The date that I will never forget. In a second, my life changes. Forever. One second, I am dribbling the ball with a smile on my face looking to pass it to my teammate. The next thing I remember is switching directions and falling to the ground in excruciating pain. I have never felt this amount of pain before. My coaches rush over as I scream in pain. I know something is wrong. Seriously wrong. My teammates look terrified as I try to grab the turf under me for any sort of support, but that support wasn't there. I feel like I will forever be stuck on the field. It was like one of those dreams where you can't move. My coach is the next thing I remember. He asked me what happened. I tried to speak, but my voice was drowning in my sobs. I told him that I felt a pop and he tells me it will be ok. I hope more than anything that I will be ok. After he looked at my knee, my coach held out his hands for me to grab onto to help me up. I grab his hands and get up. I put my arms around him and a teammate. I wonder if she will ever be my teammate again as I hobble to a golf cart that someone must have brought over. My teammates hand me my soccer bag. The man in the golf cart asks me if I am ok, but it is hard to hear him over the screams of the engine. "I am not ok," I think to myself. I'm not sure what words I actually said out loud. I text my mom, "Where are you parked? I hurt my knee really bad." My mom pulls up and I get in the car. I try to hold in my tears until the car door closes. My mom knows right away something is very wrong. I tell her everything that happened. She calls my dad and I speak with him, and he sounds so defeated. When I got home my dad meets me with crutches. He looks heartbroken. It is terrible for a father to see his child like this. I crutch upstairs and immediately cry myself to sleep.

The next day, I wake up and immediately look at my knee. I think to myself, *"Wow it is really swollen."* My left knee is almost three times larger than my other knee. I ask my mom if I can stay home from school because I can't move my leg. Luckily, she agrees. I'm icing 24/7. One thing I learn to do immediately is to ice, ice, and ice some more. Icing on the first day seems like it helps a lot with the pain. The swelling stays the same though. My dad tells me I am going to the doctor. At 2 p.m. that afternoon, I head over to UCLA to meet with the doctor. My mom, dad, and I wait sit in the waiting room until they call my name. I crutch into the room and the nurse tells me I need to get an x-ray. After my x-ray, I wait for the doctor. When the doctor arrives, he does some tests on my knee. He tells me that it might be an ACL tear and that I'll need an MRI. Even though I've been expecting to hear this, I die a little inside. After the appointment, my mom drives me home. I go to bed crying again.

The following day, I wake up and get ready for school. This is my first day back at school since my injury. I am terrified as I have no idea what to expect. My mom takes me to school early so I can ask the school for accommodations as it's difficult to get around on crutches. Happily, my school helps with this, and I head to meet my friends who are amazingly gracious to help me carry my things the entire day. My teachers agree to let me leave each class early so I can get a head start to get to my next class on time and not risk getting bumped getting to the next class. This day feels like it is going on forever. The end of day bell finally rings and that means I get to leave and go home. My mom agrees to let me hang out with my friends for a little while after school to cheer me up. I hang out with my friends for an hour or so and then head straight back to UCLA for my MRI. I am terrified.

When we arrive, they ask me to wear special clothes. I lay down and put on the headphones they give me. While I was on the MRI table, I realized I have to stay positive. No matter what the results are, I need to stay positive and never give up on getting back to soccer, getting back to who I am. The MRI lasts 15 minutes and they tell me I can go home and that I should get the results in a few days. My mom drives me home. I cry, but not as much. When we get home, I just crawl into bed and go to sleep.

I wake up. It is Saturday so I sleep in for a little bit. I ice, like it seems like I always do now and eat breakfast in bed. I'm starting to realize the swelling comes down a little when I continuously ice. It does help. I have been working on getting my range of motion back just like the doctor told me to do. I put my ankle on a hard surface so that gravity can push my leg down. It is helping a lot.

Not a lot happened today. I still haven't gotten my MRI results back yet. I am scared about what it is going to say. I feel like my world is hanging in the balance. All I do today is ice and rest and think. I have fallen into a specific schedule. I wish more than anything that I could have my old life back.

Sunday, I again slept in. Once I wake up, I immediately start icing. I have noticed that the swelling in my knee has gone down quite a bit. My doctor told me that I can't have surgery until I have good motion in my knee and the swelling goes down. To have good motion in my knee, I need to be able to completely straighten my knee and bend my knee at least 100 degrees. I have been practicing bending and straightening my knee every single day since my injury. I'm going to make this happen. My mom bought me an ice machine which is really effective for icing my knee. It is much better than a regular ice pack because I can set it to go on and off during the day or night. You can buy an ice machine on Amazon. All I do today is ice and stretch and try to stay positive. I think I can do this.

Today is a big day. This is the day that I find out my MRI results. I am so nervous. This news will determine the rest of my life. I pray that it is not torn. Deep down, I think it is torn. I would not have this amount of pain if it wasn't torn. I have to go to school today. I wonder how school is going to go. It is so tiring having to crutch around school all day. My arms have become terribly sore. On the bright side, I will likely become incredibly strong and jacked by the end of all this. I try to stay positive and find the good in this mess. As the day goes on, it feels like time is moving 10 times more slowly than usual. Every 30 minutes I text my dad asking for any news. I assume he must be extremely annoyed with my impatience. He responds with the same thing, saying there is no news. It is not until 1:45 when I receive the text from my dad that changes everything, "Avi - I just spoke to the radiologist. I'm so sorry but the ACL is torn. The other ligaments all look good. We love you, Avi. You will be back on the field at the end of the year." In that moment, my heart shattered into a million pieces. I had to try my best to not break down and cry in the middle of English class. I felt tears forming in my eyes, but I held them in. When the school bell rang, I waited for my sister to come over and we went straight to her car. I started crying. It was uncontrollable. It was like a piece of me was gone, never to return. In an attempt to make me feel better, she took me to Starbucks. You know what? It did make me feel a little bit better. When we got home, my mom told me I had to leave to go to physical therapy. I met with the physical therapist, and he helped teach me exercises to strengthen my knee. When it was over, my mom and I drove home, and I went right to my bed. I imagined my bed was a black hole and, somehow, I could crawl into it and never return to real life. It was oddly sort of comforting in such a miserable time.

The next day, I did not go to school because my knee pain was too much for me to handle. My mom has been so amazing during this time. I have learned to welcome the support of the people closest to me, rather than try to push them away. It is much easier going through this with the support of my loved ones. I try to remember that, and I hope you will as well. I spent the day icing and doing my PT exercises. It seems like an ongoing cycle: ice, PT, ice, PT, ice, PT. As I do my exercises, I work on my homework. It is incredibly important that I focus on school during this time away from soccer. To be able to go to a good college, my grades need to be just as incredible as my soccer skills. It's so easy these days to fall behind in school so please remember to keep up.

Catching up can be so difficult if you fall behind. There is not a lot more to say about this day.

Showering can be very difficult after a major knee injury. Sorry to have to tell you that. It is simply very difficult to maneuver my knee. I have learned to wake up extra early, so I have more time for stuff like this and this has helped me to have enough time to get ready for school. At school, I have to crutch around for 6 hours which is really difficult. As the days go on, I realize I am finally starting to get used to using my crutches. Hey, my arms are getting stronger so that's a positive. I learned to ask my teachers for help and tell them my situation so they will be ok with me being a few minutes late to class. Asking for help doesn't always come easy so be sure to work on that. It takes me a while to get to each class so it is a lot less stressful knowing that I can be a few minutes late to class and my teacher will understand. Because of my lack of mobility, I have to turn down a lot of offers to hang out with my friends. It is very hard to walk places with my friends. They sort of understand, but it means that I'm not spending as much time with them as I used to. I miss them. Miss them a lot.

Today is the first time I am going back to soccer practice since my injury. Not to play, of course, but just to hang out with my teammates. I know this is going to be so difficult. I am terribly sad just thinking about this. It is going to be very hard seeing my team play soccer and knowing that I will not be able to play for such a long time. When I get to practice, my teammates come up and give me a big hug. That means a lot to me. They know how sad I am, so they try to cheer me up. My coach asks me how I am doing and tries to make jokes to make me feel better. The second I see my team start to warm-up, the emotions start to kick in. I try not to cry and try to put on a brave face. I still support my teammates from the sidelines. When practice is over, one of my teammates pulls me aside and tells me she has some important news. She tells me she tore her ACL a couple of months ago and has been secretly playing on it and that her parents are ok with this. The news shocks me as I could never understand how someone could keep this news from the team just to keep playing. I know that she's risking her future health doing this, so I encourage her to tell our coach. She says she will tell him soon. I can't understand how someone could risk permanently damaging their body. My teammate tells me she is planning to have surgery in a few weeks. I can see that she loves soccer just as much as I do.

The next day I wake up to a very swollen knee which really scared me. Just getting around school made me so exhausted that I almost fell during lunch today. I realize I have to figure out how to manage my time and energy, so I have enough to get through the day. After school, I go over to my friend's house. It is nice to keep my relationships with my friends strong while I am recovering from this injury. Seeing my friends helps me stay focused and keeps me optimistic about the future. Friends are so important, especially during difficult times like this.

It's finally Saturday but this is not a good day. I am at home doing nothing while my team is out playing the sport I love, soccer, in front of college coaches at a national showcase. Today was supposed to be my chance to show college coaches what I can do on the soccer field, but instead I'm sitting on the couch watching Netflix. The hardest thing to accept is that there is nothing I can do right now to make this any better. I keep thinking of the "what if's." What if I never play soccer again? What if I never play the same? What if I never have the same love for the game? These questions keep running through my mind throughout the day. It is so difficult because every time I open my phone, I see what my teammates post about the soccer games and the showcase. I will forever think about what might have been if I hadn't hurt my knee that day at practice and, instead, I was playing in this showcase with my team.

I realized something today. My entire journey is in my hands. It is up to me to do all of my physical therapy, all of my icing, and doing whatever is best for my body. I can't defer my responsibilities to anyone else. It is my body, and I need to prioritize getting back to playing soccer. I can't cut corners because that would only hurt me. It has been hard for me to stay motivated to do anything at this point. Soccer has been a good outlet for me to stay motivated, but now I've lost that. Without soccer, I need to find new passions to keep me motivated. Since I won't be able to play soccer for a while, I need to commit my time to other things. I have started to become interested in photography and I'm taking photos of the team at our practices. I really enjoy photography. Maybe there's something there.

I am also trying to find joy in the little things. For example, I got an A on my math quiz today! These successes help distract me from thinking about my knee. My knee didn't hurt at all at school today which is amazing. I feel so upset because I found out that some people don't believe that I am that injured. I don't understand how people could believe that I would fake such a serious injury. I miss soccer more than anything. Soccer is my love.

My parents and I are debating on which type of surgery I should get. There are three types of grafts used to put the ACL back together. These three options are patella, quadriceps, and hamstring. We are leaning towards either patella or quadriceps. There are pros and cons for each type of graft. For the patella, patients say that they get pain in their kneecap after the surgery when they kneel on their knee. The quadriceps is a newer type of surgery. My teammate had the quad surgery and her recovery has been amazing. I haven't decided yet, so I am going to continue to do more research.

Today I am meeting with a new orthopedic surgeon. He did the ACL repair for one of my teammates and her recovery has been very quick. I have to wake up very early and I am going to miss school for the beginning of the school day. When I meet him, I get a gut feeling telling me he is going to be the doctor for me. He is extremely nice and made me feel so comfortable asking questions. He checks my knee and tells me that I am ready for surgery which is such a great thing to hear after all of my hard work. They schedule me for April 26 and I immediately start counting down the days.

It's Saturday so I don't have school today, which is really nice. I get to sleep in. My dad bought me a slant pillow for my bed which helps keep my leg elevated while I sleep. My doctor said it is best to keep my leg elevated to help the swelling go down. Some good news is that I had to get a smaller brace because my leg is now too small for the brace I got right after my injury. That is a good sign because it means my swelling has gone down a lot.

In exactly 10 days, I'm having surgery on my ACL. I am both excited and nervous because you never know what can happen during surgery. I am confident that I will be ok because I trust my surgeon.

Coachella is today, which is very exciting. It also reminds me that I can't go to concerts and other things like that because of my knee. That thought saddens me. My favorite artist, Harry Styles, performed last night so I stayed up late to watch the live stream. It was one of the most incredible performances I have ever seen in my entire life. I wish I had been there in person.

Just nine days until my surgery. It is weird not having anything to do on the weekend. Usually, I would be at a soccer game or soccer showcase. It doesn't help knowing there are so many things I am missing out on. My doctor says I will miss at least a week of school after my surgery, so I need to make sure I keep up with my schoolwork.

Today I was really unproductive which is not good for my recovery. I woke up extremely late. Skipping meals is also not good for my recovery. My recovery is entirely up to me, and if I decide to be lazy, I will never get back to the level I was playing at before my injury. I am terrified that the surgery will go wrong, and I will never fully recover. My dad has been amazing as he has done hours of research to make sure my recovery is successful.

I'm trying to stay focused on practical day-to-day things. For example, I found that constantly using my ice machine is so important. This is why my swelling has gone down so much. The machine keeps my knee cold for hours and hours.

Today my family and I played the game "Taboo." I was on a team with my mom and my sister was on a team with my dad. I love playing games. That is one of the reasons I love soccer so much. I love any competition and soccer is all competition. We ended up tying, but I like to think that my mom and I won. After the game, I Facetimed one of my best friends just to catch up with her. Whenever I am sad about anything I call her, and she makes everything better. We talk for a while until my mom makes me hang up and go to bed.

I am going to watch my team practice today. I am really excited to see my friends and teammates again because they are one of my main sources of happiness at this current moment. Before I get to leave, my mom makes me clean my room and do all of my jobs. For as long as I can remember, my mom always makes me do my chores before I am allowed to go to any place. I think she does this to make sure I learn responsibility and learn how to be accountable for my jobs. I am grateful that my mom has instilled these values into my mind so that I can be a better person because of her.

Today I am focusing on catching up on my homework. I need to make sure that I don't get behind on my work. Especially since I'm having surgery soon, I need to get ahead on my homework, so I don't have to worry about it after surgery when I am in an extreme amount of pain. One assignment is to write an essay about something about which I am extremely passionate. I got a lot of my research done which is really important to me. I want to get the hard parts completed so I don't have to concern myself with them after my surgery.

I am so excited that I am getting my surgery in 3 days. Today I am going to start setting goals for myself. I am going to try and bend my knee 130 degrees before my surgery. I am at 125 degrees so I am trying to get the extra 5 degrees so I can be even more prepared for surgery. It is really good for me to get my leg as mobile as possible before my surgery so that the rehab after surgery will be a lot easier. I can now completely straighten my knee which is really good for my mobility. Each day I am going to continue to bend it a little bit more until I reach my goal.

Tomorrow is my surgery day and I can hardly wait. I go to school and look forward to the final bell letting me know that I can finally go home. When I go home, I go straight to my room. I am so nervous I can't even speak to anyone. I work really hard on my PT exercises so my knee will be in as good shape as possible going for tomorrow. I have to sleep downstairs after the surgery because I will not be able to walk up the stairs. I set up where I am going to sleep and make sure I have everything I need for tomorrow morning. I go to bed early so I will get plenty of sleep.

SURGERY

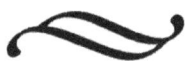

Today is surgery day! I am equally excited and terrified. I wake up at 5:30 a.m. and get ready to head to the hospital. My mom and dad drive me to Santa Monica, and we arrive at 7:00 a.m. When I get taken in, I change into a gown and lay down. Multiple doctors and nurses come in and talk to me about my surgery. A nurse comes in and puts in my IV. Surprisingly, it did not hurt at all. I wait for about 45 minutes until a doctor comes in and tells me I am ready for surgery. They give me an injection and also a nerve blocker into my leg. I immediately feel the effects of the sedative and they wheel me into the operating room. I don't remember much after that. The next thing I know, I am waking up in a new room. When I wake up, my parents walk into the room and say hello to me. I feel incredibly sleepy and a little nauseous. I am told that is a result of the anesthesia. After a couple of hours, they tell me I am free to go home. A guy enters the room with a wheelchair for me. My parents help me into the wheelchair and he wheels me to my mom's car. I fall asleep for most of the car ride home. When I get home, I immediately go to sleep for the rest of the night.

The day after surgery, I wake up with an incredible amount of pain in my knee. It is excruciating. My mom finds me awake and she gives me medication. I switch off between icing, doing PT, and sleeping. I also cry a lot. I feel extremely defeated already. My mom tries to help with words of encouragement. I try to complete my PT exercises. It is really difficult for me. My leg feels extremely weak. My mom has to help me every time I have to go to the bathroom. I am extremely exhausted just going to the bathroom. A lot of my friends reach out to me, which is so nice to hear. It helps knowing that people care about me during this difficult time.

Today is the same as yesterday, I wake up and complete my PT exercises. It is still extremely difficult which is so upsetting. When I am not doing PT, I am icing at all times to help the swelling go down. I still feel extremely fatigued. I can't manage to straighten my leg while lifting it up no matter how hard I try. Such a simple movement is now a challenge. Any confidence that I ever had is gone due to my lack of mobility. I take a break and go to sleep. When I wake up from my nap, I try my exercises again. It is difficult to exercise through my tears. There are many parts of me that want to throw in the towel and give up, but I think about how amazing it will be once I get back on the soccer field. That keeps me motivated.

Three days after surgery; I feel like I will never be the same player I was. This is miserable. I have never been in so much pain in my entire life. I feel weak and useless. I have cried every single day since my surgery. The hours pass by and all I do is just lie down and do nothing. This feels like torture. My mom is doing her best to help me do basic functions like go to the bathroom and get dressed and I am so grateful for her. She is making this process a little bit easier. Today I am starting my first day with my new physical therapist. This is the first time since I had surgery that I am leaving my house. I am terrified that I am going to hurt my knee somehow and this whole process will be all for nothing.

Today is exactly a month since I tore my ACL. It is crazy to think that only a month ago I was able to play the sport that I love more than anything. A part of me is scared that I am going to lose my passion for soccer throughout my long recovery. It is scary to consider that maybe soccer will never be the same once I get healthy again. One amazing achievement is that I can complete leg lifts easily. I couldn't do this at all right after surgery and now, just four days later, I am seeing some progress. It is really great to see my hard work paying off, even if it is a small achievement.

Today is my brother's birthday. I feel bad that because of me, my family and I can't do activities today that I could normally do. I am not able to do a lot of things I could normally do and it makes me sad knowing I might never be the same person I was before all of this. I am starting to feel like the days are all blending together. I feel as though I am living in one long nightmare in which I keep experiencing my worst fears over and over again. Even though I am doing well in physical therapy, I do not feel I am improving enough.

Today I woke up and went to physical therapy. My physical therapist told me that I am making lots of progress. I was able to lay on my side and lift my leg up and down without any pain. My PT had me use a "Russian Stem" machine which helps activate my quad muscles while I do my exercises. By the time I was done, I could activate my quadriceps muscle more than when I started. I felt really confident when I left my appointment. When I got home, I had a lack of energy and decided to take a nap. I have learned to know when my body needs a break.

I am finally going to see my surgeon to see how my recovery is going so far. We have an hour's drive down to Santa Monica. When I arrive, they take x-rays of my knee. Then, I went back to meet my doctor. When he comes in, he asks me to take off my brace so he can see the progress I am making. He takes off my brace and the ace bandage under. It is the first time since my surgery that I have seen my knee. I was extremely nervous to see my knee because I was worried there would be something wrong. Luckily, my doctor said my knee looked perfectly fine and said I am actually ahead of schedule.

This morning, I went to PT again and did my regular exercises. My PT told me that I am doing really well and that it is obvious that I have been practicing a lot outside of PT. After I got home from PT, I was really happy when my friend's parents brought over a care package for me. It was the first time someone had brought me a gift since my surgery and it felt really nice knowing someone cared.

Believe it or not, today is the first time since my surgery that I am actually going to take a full shower. I am very nervous because I can't get my knee wet. My mom has to help me get into the shower and take off my brace. It takes a long time to actually shower and I realize this is how my life is going to be for a long time. It is scary thinking how much I am going to have to adjust my lifestyle after my surgery. After my shower I go to bed because just showering takes a lot of energy out of me. I have to learn to preserve my energy.

Last night, I was finally able to get some quality sleep, which is a huge relief. When I wake up, my mom tells me I have to study for my French quiz. I have a lot of tests and quizzes to make up when I return to school. I study for many hours until I notice it is dark out. I am starting to notice the days are passing by a lot more quickly than usual. I love that I don't have to go through anything alone because my parents are extremely involved in my life. I am very blessed.

Today is Mother's Day and I am excited that I get to celebrate my mother today. My mother has done so much for me throughout the years and she deserves all of the praise given. My sister plans for a fun day for us to do. It might be difficult with my knee to do everything she has planned, which is really disappointing. Afterwards, we hang out for the rest of the day and it is really fun!

I had a phone call with a very special person today. I still can't believe I was lucky enough to have a phone call with him. He gave me an amazing piece of advice that I will forever keep in my mind. He said after his own surgery he realized that there are two types of pain. The pain you have before surgery when it is only getting worse and the pain you get after surgery when you are getting better. I have to know that pain is normal during recovery and that some days are going to be worse than others. I can't let the fear of pain stop me from getting better. This advice really helps me keep a positive mindset.

Today I can bend my knee up to 70 degrees which is great for just 2 weeks since surgery. According to my doctor's plan, I should be at 90 degrees by 4 weeks. Pretty soon, I will be able to walk without crutches. First, I will need to get used to using one crutch and then move to no crutches. I am going to attend practice today for my team's tryouts; not to play, of course, but at least I can hang out with the team. This helps me feel like I'm still a part of the team. There were a lot of new girls trying out and it is making me nervous to think I won't have a spot next year because I am injured.

Today is the second day of my team's tryouts. I've been acting as the unofficial photographer for the team as a way to contribute to my team while I can't play on the field. I am starting to get the hang of it, but I am still pretty new at this. My mom says it is good for me to stay involved with my team, but it makes me feel even worse seeing what I am missing out on. On a lighter note, I can finally bend my knee a little bit further! It feels good to have these little accomplishments. At tryouts, I talked with one of my teammates who also went through ACL surgery. She gives me a lot of advice, which is really helpful. One thing she told me is that recovery is like a rollercoaster. There are ups and downs and you never know what is going to happen, but everything will turn out ok in the end.

I do not have anything to do today which is both good and bad. That means that I can focus on doing my

PT. I am working on putting more weight on my injured leg while still using my crutches. I can't get rid of the crutches yet because I also tore my meniscus. One thing I've learned that is important for recovery is to make sure you are eating right. Nutrition is a huge part of the recovery process. If you eat badly, your body won't heal right, and you will weaken over time.

Today I learned a big lesson about icing. I was not smart and I didn't ice all morning. Now it is hard for me to get my range of motion. I can only bend it to 50 degrees where I was bending to 70 degrees. I will keep trying throughout the day, but I know now I have to keep icing at all times. My parents and doctors are saying I can finally go back to school on Monday. I am so excited to finally get to see my friends again. I know it is going to be a big adjustment getting used to going to school again.

Today is the first time I am seeing my team play in a game since my injury. I am very excited to take pictures of my team playing with my new camera. I am happy to be involved in the game without being on the field. Another thing that is exciting is that my high school soccer coach called me yesterday to check up on me. He wanted to let me know that he wants me to be a captain and be a huge part of the team. It makes me feel really good to know that someone cares about my recovery and wants to check in on me. After my team's game I felt completely exhausted. It was a little sad thinking about all the games I am going to miss over the next year.

START OF RECOVERY

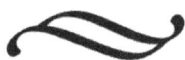

Today is my first day back to school since my surgery! I have mixed feelings about finally returning. On one hand, I am so thrilled to see my friends again after a long time. At the same time, I am absolutely terrified that something awful will happen. Specifically, I am scared of injuring myself and making this whole journey for nothing. I am also scared that I will be miserable at school. It will be hard getting used to being at school after staying at home for almost a month.

By the time the day ends, I am completely exhausted. My body is not used to being active for six plus hours. When I get home, I take a nap for the majority of the afternoon. It will take a lot of effort to get used to going to school.

I am about one month out from surgery, and it still feels weird to think I had surgery. My knee doesn't hurt as much as it did, but I still can't do much on it. It is kind of difficult seeing how much fun my teammates are having on the field. I am thankful I am not a junior because if I were, I would have no shot of getting recruited to play soccer in college. I hope that I become even stronger after this. That's what my teammates say usually happens.

Flash forward. It's the second to last day of school. I never thought this day would come! This year has been extremely difficult for me because of my knee injury. Nonetheless, I managed to maintain good grades and still had a good experience during my sophomore year. My school and teachers have been so amazing in helping me get through this school year.

I am so happy today. Today is my sister's high school graduation! She has worked so hard and I am excited to see her walk in her graduation. Even though I don't typically have to wear my knee brace anymore, I wear it today because the graduation is very crowded and I don't want to risk injuring my knee. It is uncomfortable wearing the brace, but it is more important to keep my knee safe, even if that means being uncomfortable for a couple of hours.

Even though its summer, I still have work to do. Every Monday and Wednesday, I go to PT for one hour each time. I am slowly starting to enjoy PT because I am finally getting into a routine. I start each session by doing

15 minutes on the stationary bike. Then, I do different range-of-motion exercises to get my leg stretched out. After that, I do "BFR" which is meant to make me feel as if I am doing 3 exercises at once, if that makes sense. I put on a band on the top of my leg and when the machine turns on, it cuts off my blood flow so each exercise I do is even more difficult. After that, I do balance work and then the hour is over. After PT, icing is important.

Today is Father's Day and I love Father's Day because it is a great reminder that I have such a great dad who is always there to help me. I wake up early and get ready to go to brunch with my family. I wear jeans instead of shorts because I am extremely scared that my knee will get sunburned and then my scars might never heal correctly. It is annoying that I have to wear jeans especially because it is almost 100 degrees outside. Still, I have an amazing time spending time with my family on such a special day. One tip I have learned is to place silicone strips on top of my scars as that helps lighten and heal the scars.

I am very proud of myself as I can finally notice visible improvement in PT. At first, I was discouraged as I could barely see any improvements. Now, I can finally start seeing my knee gaining muscle definition and strength. I can bend 140 degrees which is so nice when I look at the numbers. Still, I have good days and very bad days. The most important thing besides PT is what I do after. After each PT session, I make sure to ice A LOT so my knee can recover after each tough session. Each time I go to PT, it gets more intense as I keep improving. So, it is very necessary to take care of my body every day as it is so important to keep getting stronger.

I am also trying to get back into reading books and to stop using my phone as much. I have noticed that the more I use my phone, the more tired I become. Since it is summer, I am focusing on reading summer-themed books! My club soccer team is coming back from break, so I finally get to go back to practice again. When I went to PT, I passed a soccer ball with my physical therapist for the first time since I tore my ACL. It was such a weird experience touching a soccer ball again. Sometimes I thought I would never kick a soccer ball again, so it was so amazing that I accomplished that.

It is officially 100 days since I tore my ACL. It feels like it happened such a long time ago. I honestly can't remember my life before my injury, which is upsetting. I am so excited because I just got invited to my teammate's birthday party. I am mainly happy because she invited me even though I'm injured which means she is still thinking about me even though I'm not at games and practices like usual. We are all going to the beach. I haven't gone swimming since my injury, and I am thrilled to be moving back into my normal life.

Tonight, I am going to a concert with my entire family. It is going to be difficult because I am going to be surrounded by a lot of people and hope I don't get injured. There is always a possibility that someone will accidently bump into me and hurt my knee. I remind myself that, even though I got injured, I can't live the rest of my life fearing getting hurt. I'm so glad I went as the concert was absolutely incredible and I had a fantastic time hanging out with my family. The music was amazing and so was the atmosphere. When I was there, time stopped, and I was just living in the moment.

Today I am going to that really good friend's birthday party! The plan is for us to go to the beach for a while. The problem is I am not allowed to go in the ocean because of my knee. So, I will be stuck sitting on the beach while everyone hangs out in the water. That part won't be fun but, honestly, I am just happy to be included!

I have been talking to my high school coach lately. It is important for me to stay in contact with my coach, so he doesn't forget about me. We have been talking about next season and he wants to know my goals that I have for the team. I don't know if I will be able to play in time for next season, but I might have a shot but if I keep working hard on a consistent basis.

The one thing I am really stressed about is college recruiting. There are so many things that stress me out, such as if I have enough time or will they even want me if I'm injured. I am scared that when I do come back, I won't have enough time to get recruited and my whole soccer life has been for nothing. If that happens, it will feel like I wasted my whole childhood for nothing. It doesn't help that it feels like all of my teammates are getting committed to play in college while I am stuck being injured.

AHHHHH!!! Tomorrow my family is heading to Pismo Beach for our annual family vacation. I haven't packed yet, so I really need to do that. I always have trouble packing. I either overpack or underpack and forget everything important. This year is different because of my knee. I need to pack all of my physical therapy equipment. Hopefully, this year will still be fun despite the circumstances.

It is the first day of vacation! My family wants to do all of these activities like hiking and going into the ocean. I know it isn't intentional, but I sort of feel left out. I obviously am not allowed to hike or go in the ocean because I am still rehabbing my knee. Part of me is apprehensive about going on vacation because I am worried about being left out. I cannot wait until my knee has healed!

Despite the limitations from my knee, I am having so much fun in Pismo Beach. Everything is amazing. My family is getting along so well, and I never want to go back home. The weather here is perfect. I brought my physical therapy equipment to Pismo Beach so I can keep up with my exercises. My family and I have decided to watch a new movie together every night. Last night we watched the movie Father of the Bride. My dad was so emotional that he cried!!!!!

Since getting home from vacation, I have been working on my photography and videography to help give me a focus while I can't play soccer. They are both really fun but, obviously, I want to be on the field again. On the other hand, PT is going well. I am creating so many good relationships there and I love being there. I enjoy going to PT and that is so great! I get along so well with my physical therapist and that is such an important relationship for my recovery to be successful.

THE LONG HAUL

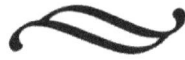

I went to school to pick up my books for the upcoming school year which was a huge reminder that summer is almost over. I also took my school picture. I was so nervous about the photo. After it was over, I felt very relieved.

PT is getting so fun! Now that I am improving, I can actually do exercises that I truly enjoy. I am even sweating again which shows I am working hard. There was a certain point in time where I actually disliked going to PT. That sounds bad, but I felt like I wasn't making any progress and I hated being there as it just reminded me of how far away from returning to soccer I was. Now, I feel myself making significant progress and feel motivated again. This reminds me that I need to stay consistent no matter the circumstances, because you never know when you will make a breakthrough. Consistency is so important.

School is slowly approaching, and I am trying to get the most out of summer before it is over. I finally saw my friends again! It has been hard for all of us to hang out because we all have such busy schedules. So, it is so amazing when I get to see them every so often. Today was so much fun with them. We just drive around and blast music. It is so much fun, and I feel genuinely happy for a couple of hours.

AHHHH!! Tomorrow is the first day of school! All I can think about are all the things that could possibly go wrong. What if I can't find my classes? What if I fall down in front of everyone? What if I hurt my knee? Every time I think of school, I get this giant pit in my stomach. It is so bad that I can't even fall asleep. I stay up most of the night stressed out about school. I try so hard to fall asleep, but without much success. I am wide awake most of the night.

Finally, it's Saturday! What an amazing day! I get to hang out with my friends all day! I think today was the perfect day. First of all, my friends and I drove around, which is seriously the best thing you can ever do. Also, we watched funny videos and old Disney movies. After that, we ordered some food and just talked for hours. I had so much fun and wouldn't have chosen anything better. I didn't want the night to ever be over, but all good things must come to an end. Otherwise, how can you ever have better things happen to you?

I had my first quiz of the school year today. I felt so confident going into it because I studied super hard all night. It feels so good when all your hard work pays off. I am so excited to see if I got a good grade on the quiz! After school, I quickly finished my homework so I could go to my practice. I haven't been to practice in a long time, so it is good to be there again. Hopefully, just like with my schoolwork, all of my hard work in physical therapy will pay off when I get to finally play soccer again.

I am working really hard to finish all of my upcoming homework so I can have time to hang out with my friends this week. I am taking really difficult, time-consuming classes so I try to take advantage of every opportunity where I can get ahead on my work. This year, my classes are going to be very difficult. This is also the perfect time to get ahead on my schoolwork. I finally finished late tonight and went right to sleep. I was so excited that I could focus on spending time with my friends instead of having to do homework.

I'm kind of nervous for school tomorrow because my knee feels so tight after a long day of school. I talked to my PT and asked what would help with this. He told me to stretch my leg out consistently throughout the day. He says it would also help if I could prop my leg up to keep it straight during class. I am going to start doing this and hopefully it will significantly help. I'm glad I told my PT about this and asked for help, which is another thing I've learned to do to help with my recovery.

OMG OMG OMG!!!! I just made a big step. Today at practice, I warmed up with my team! That may sound insignificant, but that is such a big deal for me. I got to run and stretch with my team for the first time since my injury. I cried when I was warming up, just because I was so proud of myself. I'm not at the stage when I can fully practice yet, but it is really good that I can visibly see my progress. I can't wait until I can practice at the level I know I can. My coach watched me warm up and was so happy for me!!

Today I had the hardest PT session ever. When it was done, I was literally dripping with sweat. I ran so much and practiced a lot with the ball. I was really proud of myself mainly because, until today, I was not confident I could do any of those exercises. I was so surprised to be able to sprint so fast, but it felt amazing in the moment. When it was over, I felt so good about myself. I truly haven't felt like that since I tore my ACL. My PT also told me that he was so proud of my progress.

I am so nervous for tomorrow. I have a very important class essay in IB History of the Americas. For the essay, I can't use any notes. All I can do is study and hope that I can write a good solid essay in only 45 minutes. All day, I have been studying with my mom. I have been going over all of my notes until they are completely engraved into my mind. I can't stop thinking about how tomorrow is going to go. Hopefully, all my hard work will pay off and I will do well.

This weekend, I am watching the University of Michigan football game with my family. This player named Ronnie Bell just came back from an ACL injury and his story is really inspiring. It really makes me feel better seeing someone have such a successful recovery. When I watch him play, it doesn't even seem like he was ever injured. Sometimes when I think about my recovery, it makes me less anxious when I watch someone in the same situation as me. All I need to do is take my recovery one day at a time and have tunnel vision towards the end goal.

Football Sunday is a very big deal in my family. I am also doing a fantasy football league in my Broadcasting class. I love healthy competition, so I am so excited for this! I think I have a very good team this year so I can't wait. I am a very competitive person, and I haven't had an outlet for my competitiveness since tore my ACL. Fantasy football is a really good way for me to be competitive in a safe way. I can't wait!

Guess what!!!!! I am sprinting! Can you even believe it? A couple of months ago I wouldn't have imagined that I would be doing anything like this ever again. It feels so amazing to actually sweat again. I seriously can't believe I just wrote that sentence. I never realized how amazing it is to work out. I missed this for so long and now that I can do this again, it feels like a dream. That is the only way to describe this. Also, my birthday is in exactly one week and I am so excited to finally be 17 years old.

I think the hardest part of this journey is how long it is. Sometimes I feel like I am making such an improvement, but then I think about how much longer I have until I will be able to play again. That makes me feel so defeated. My mom taught me a good piece of advice that helps me stay motivated. She told me to set small goals instead of one large goal so that I have good steppingstones to follow until I am able to play again. For example, those goals can be beginning to run, sprinting, and getting to pass. Instead of just looking towards returning to play, achieving small goals will help keep you motivated to get to that big goal in the end.

Today I am filming the Homecoming game. Our football team is extremely good this year, so it is always fun to see them play. I am live streaming the game for people who are unable to go see the game in person, so I have to make sure the experience is a good one. The one bad part is my feet get so tired because I am standing for such long periods of time. One good part is I get a really good view of the game because I am on the roof of the press box. We ended up winning 55-0 and it was such a great game to watch.

It's football Sunday again! I love this day because it is such a fun day no matter what is happening. Everyone in my family gathers in the family room to watch whatever football game is on. It is the one time a week where everyone is doing the same thing despite our busy schedules. We all love watching football because we all truly love the game. Our favorite team is the Washington Commanders. They may not be the best team in the league, but we all root for them, win or lose. It is important for families to have common interests.

Today is my birthday!!!!!!!! I am so happy! This is my special day! I am turning 17 years old today. I can't believe I am 17. It feels like yesterday that I was turning 14. That is the weird thing about this time. Time feels so weird and fast. I still feel like I am in 2019 and am still in 8th grade. But surprisingly, I'm a junior in high school and am growing up so fast. Growing up is so scary because you can't stop it or slow it down. You just have to accept growing up and changing.

I am so sad today because my dog is very sick. His heart is failing, and he is really struggling. Every day, we have to give him tons of pills so he can stay alive. He hates taking the pills, but he always does because I think he knows he needs them. It's crazy that, even though he is a dog, he knows deep down what is best for him. I love my dog so much. As much as I hate dealing with my

ACL, I hate that my dog also is going through medical issues. I wish we weren't going through this together.

I just had two hours of physical therapy and I am so drained. I feel so weak and tired, but I know it is going to help me in the long run. It has been such a long time since I have pushed myself past my limits in a workout. I still have so much homework left to do tonight. I don't know how I am going to balance all of this work when I can finally play again. I am working to improve my time management skills so I can establish good habits for the future.

I filmed the football game again tonight. This time, I got to be on the field and film. While I was filming, I realized that this may be what I want to do for the rest of my life. I love broadcasting. I had so much fun, and I felt so comfortable doing it. Usually, I feel uncomfortable in these types of public situations, but I was having way too much fun to even worry about that. I genuinely want to do this as a career, and I am so happy that I found my passion so early. I love sports and I love broadcasting so sports broadcasting is the perfect career for me.

PROGRESS:
SLOWLY BUT SURELY

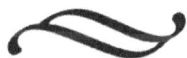

While I've been recovering from my ACL surgery, I have been using this time to create my highlight reel to send to college coaches. I hope this will help them get an idea of the kind of player I am. I am still worried that they won't be interested in me if I've been injured. Everyone around me says I have so much time, but what if I don't? I am nervous to email college coaches.

Physical therapy was so good today! I am finally jumping with my left leg. A couple of weeks ago, I had no ability to even attempt to jump on my left foot. Now I have strengthened my leg a ton. I am so happy with my progress thus far. I am starting to feel like myself again and I am so excited to keep progressing.

Today I went for my return-to-play evaluation. Obviously, I am not close to playing again, but my surgeon wants me to get a good idea of where I am in my recovery. My mom and I have to drive all the way to downtown LA which is so far away. When I get there, I have to do a bunch of tests to compare my left leg and right leg. I am so nervous because what if I am completely behind schedule? Luckily, the PT told me that I did great, and I am ahead of schedule. Personally, I think I could have done better, but that is just because of how competitive I am.

I went on a run with my dad today. I am very excited to get back into running again. I used to love running and I love doing it again. My dad struggled to keep up with me, but he doesn't want to admit it. I forgot how good it feels to run again and I can't wait to make it a consistent thing again. My knee felt really solid which is one thing I was worried about. I was happily surprised that it felt completely normal to run. It felt like a huge weight was lifted off my shoulders. And it's good to have another fun activity to share with my dad.

Happy Thanksgiving! This is one of my favorite holidays because it is just so positive and a fun day to give thanks to everything important in my life. I am so thankful for my family for helping support me through this tough journey. I know for a fact that I would not be in the same position if I didn't have the support system that I have. I have an amazing life and I do not for a second take it for granted.

One thing I've learned through recovering from my injury that is helping me with other areas of my life is time and work management. When I have a big project that seems overwhelming, I break it up into little parts. For example, if I have an important test to study for, I will study a little each day instead of waiting until the night before to cram all the information in at once. I find myself doing better on those tests when I break it up into little sections. This tricks my mind into thinking it is easier even though I am studying the same amount for about the same amount of time. This is a better and smarter way to get tough things done.

It's almost the end of the year and I'm starting to look back and reflect on everything that has happened. This year was very hard for me and has really made me question many things in my life. There were moments where I wanted to quit because this recovery was too hard, and I felt helpless. I am so glad that I pushed through those thoughts. I proved to myself that I have so much strength inside of me. This process has made me so much stronger. I am excited for what next year has in store, and I hope that it will be a better year overall for me.

Have I mentioned how much I love Fridays? They are by far the best day of the week. Since I don't have practice on Fridays, I use this day as a day to work on my fitness. That means going on runs, hill sprints, or going on the bike. I like starting out the weekend feeling productive and knowing I'm making good choices to help with my ACL recovery.

I am really sad because my club soccer team is in Tennessee for a soccer showcase without me. I am feeling like I am missing crucial moments. Most of my teammates are seniors so I don't have that much time left with them. I have played with these girls for many years, and I want to play with them again so badly. I miss being at practice and feeling so happy with my second family. I won't be able to see them until next year due to the break for high school season, so it is going to feel like I missed so much.

Happy New Year! For this year, I am going to live life with a better attitude and outlook on life. I need to start focusing on what is best for me in life. I feel like my future will be determined by how I act in these next couple of months. I need to do well in school, soccer, and act like an adult. This year is scary because I am turning

18 this year. This means I am going to be an adult and I need to start behaving like one. Time is moving so fast, and I can't believe my teenage years are passing so quickly.

The weirdest thing is that my favorite artist is now working with my dad's favorite artist. I am talking about Taylor Swift and Aaron Dessner. This has become an important way that I can connect with my dad and have something in common with him. It is very important to find unique ways to connect with important people in your life, especially your family. Strengthening bonds is necessary to have a support system around you.

High school soccer season has officially started! It has been pre-season but now that the actual season has started, it is my favorite part of the year. I am sad, though, because I know it is going to go by too fast and then I am going to have to wait all year until I can play with my high school team again. I won't be cleared in time to play this season, so I won't be able to play again with the seniors from my school. I literally felt crushed when my doctor told me the news. I tried so hard not to cry at that moment. I am missing out on so much.

I am continuing to practice my technical skills every day so that I can be the best player I can be when I return to soccer. I am worried that I won't be at the level of my teammates. I worry that when I do come back, they will be light years ahead of me based on their skill. When I got hurt, I was at the top of my game, which was one of the most frustrating parts. I had worked so hard to raise my fitness and skill level and then I got hurt. I am doing everything I can to get back to the player I used to be.

I am starting to go on more and more runs every single day to get back in shape before I go back to club practice. I know that high school season is almost complete, and I need to start focusing on getting recruited and taking back control of my future. This means I can't get distracted. My one focus from now on must be soccer and school. If I keep focused on those two things, I can hopefully achieve my goals which don't seem so impossible anymore. My goal of returning to play is getting closer each day.

I am really sad that my high school team didn't make the playoffs. I was hoping to have more time with this team because I love them so much. I am going to miss all of the seniors because I was so close to all of them, and I never got to play on the field with them again. It is so sad to think that I will only have one more season of high school soccer. It is scary because this season went by so fast, so it is going to be the same next year. I don't want to say goodbye to this team, and I am scared at how fast time is going by.

Since high school season is over, that means my club team is resuming soon. My club team starts practicing in eleven days and I am very nervous. When we come back, I am going to be able to actually start practicing and that is very surreal. I haven't seen my team in so long and I am nervous to get back into the rhythm of playing. My knee is feeling strong, so I think the main thing is my mentality. I need to get my confidence back and become the player I used to be again. Right now, I am working on getting back in shape, so I am going on more runs and practicing more and more.

A college coach emailed me for the first time! They say they saw me play and reached out to recruit me! This is really exciting because this shows that, despite my injury, maybe I am good enough to play in college. I don't know yet if I want to go to this particular college, but it is so amazing and surreal to happen for the first time. I was starting to be worried that I was not going to be able to play at the collegiate level. I showed the email to my parents, and they were so proud of me. I can't wait for more schools to email me!

I emailed back the college coach that contacted me. I worked with my mom to write the email and I was so nervous to send it, but it felt so amazing once I had sent it. I am so excited to hopefully get a response. I did a lot of research on the college, and it does seem to be a great fit for me! I ultimately want to be a sports broadcaster or journalist and it has a really respected journalism program that would help me to accomplish my dreams.

The coach responded to me right away and asked to meet over zoom. This is all happening so fast, and I can't believe that this is even real. It has always been my dream to play soccer in college and I am so happy that all of this is happening to me right now. I don't want to jinx this, so I am not going to get my hopes up. I have never directly talked to a college coach before, so I am nervous that I am going to screw up my chance. Hopefully, everything goes well, and I can go to the college for an in-person visit.

I have been going on runs almost every single day and I realized that listening to music helps me run faster and better. When I listen to music, I feel like I forget I am running, and I do so much better. I don't know the science behind it, but it works so well, and I realized it is the key for me to run well. I feel like every time I run, I do better and better. I still have so much more to do for me to get back into soccer shape, but I definitely see the improvement. I feel myself improving my stamina and overall speed.

I finally practiced for the first time at club practice since my injury. It felt so weird but also felt so amazing at the same time. I definitely need to improve my fitness because I was not in the same shape I was before. I didn't expect myself to be perfectly fine right away, but it is still a big wake-up call that this journey is not over yet. It was amazing to see my team again, but it did not feel the same as it used to be for some reason. I can't explain it. I just wish I never went through this.

I have practice again tonight, but I am worried about playing on wet grass because it is raining where my practice is. I don't know if it is a better idea to go to practice or stay home and not risk hurting my knee in the wet area. Since tearing my ACL, I have only played on dry grass so this will be new for me, and I am a little nervous to be honest. I just need to push through my fear and play because I'm going to have to practice in the rain eventually. It might as well be now rather than later.

SETBACK

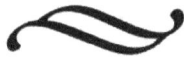

Everything has started to go so well and I'm excited to actually be able to start participating at practice. Finally, I feel like things are getting back on track. But, today at practice, I was kicking long balls with my teammate. Everything felt normal until it didn't. I was about to kick the ball and, as I planted my left foot, I felt a pop in my knee. I tried to pretend everything was fine, but I knew it wasn't. I could barely move. I was scared as I knew this feeling so well. The last time I felt something like that was when I tore my ACL. I held back the tears as I walked over to the sideline. I told my coach that my knee was hurting, and I waited until practice was over. When my dad picked me up, I didn't tell him what had happened. I refused to think that it was real. I didn't tell anyone until the next morning when I woke up and I couldn't move. My parents scheduled an MRI as soon as possible. The test came back and said everything looked fine. My surgeon told me everything looked good and just to take it easy for a bit and give my body some additional time.

I was relieved I didn't tear my ACL again. I pulled back on going to soccer practice and just focused on physical therapy. Everything was improving until, one day at PT, I put on a resistance band around my legs to start a warm-up exercise. The second I took a step, my knee completely gave out. I couldn't move. I was really scared because I could no longer straighten my knee. My mom rushed me to an orthopedic urgent care center where they took x-rays and started the process of getting yet another MRI for me.

During the days I waited to get the MRI, I pretty much already knew something was seriously wrong with my knee. After all this time, I've learned to listen to my body.

When we got the results of the MRI, the bad news was that I had torn my meniscus. This was my worst fear coming true. Hearing this confirmed was one of the worst feelings in my life. It felt like all the work and PT from the last year were for nothing. And, since my surgeon was on an extended trip out-of-town, I also had to find a new doctor. This entire experience was so scary.

My new doctor explained that I had to have surgery right away or I could permanently damage my knee. Just two days later, I was in the operating room again. After the surgery, my doctor gave us some more bad news. While my knee was open so he could repair my meniscus, he inspected my ACL and saw I had barely any of the ACL graft left. This means I need another ACL surgery. It feels like all of the work I put in this last year was for nothing. I can't believe I am going to have to do this all over again. This is all so exhausting.

Now that it's clear I need to have my ACL repaired again, we are doing a lot of research into surgeons and the best type of surgery. The biggest question is what surgeon we should pick. This choice is very important as it has to go well in order to make sure my knee is ever going to get better. We have narrowed the choices down to two options and it is very hard to pick which one because they are both great surgeons. I keep going back and forth and the decision feels almost impossible. I realize I must go with my gut on this. I have been stressing for weeks over which option I should go with for this next surgery.

I realize that I am having to spend yet another summer either doing physical therapy or icing. I am going to miss my last summer of high school trying to fix my knee instead of being a normal teenager. It is really upsetting but I know it is ultimately more important to make sure I stay healthy for the long-term. I realize I am having to sacrifice a lot due to my knee problems. I can't see my friends, go to the beach, or do normal teenage activities. I am basically going to be in my house all summer and this is my last summer until I'm an adult.

With my third knee surgery coming up, I am starting to realize that I won't be able to have a normal senior year of high school like I always dreamed of having. I won't be able to go to my senior homecoming or do senior sunrise. Will I be able to go to football games as a senior? My knee has taken so much from me, and it feels like I will never be "normal" again. I took being healthy for granted and didn't realize what I was going to lose until right now. I just wish I could have a normal senior year without worrying about hurting my knee again.

For the longest time I have seen the same physical therapist and that has meant that I was comfortable with him. All of a sudden, I have to start working with a new physical therapist, which is a big change for me. My PT is getting busier and busier, and he can't always see me. The new PT is very nice, but I sometimes struggle with getting used to new people. I was shocked when I immediately got used to seeing the new PT and it shows that I have the ability to evolve and gain new abilities.

My new dog named Luca is literally the most amazing thing to happen to our family. He is amazing at calming my other dog Zoey. When Zoey gets agitated, Luca seems to always calm her down and make her happier. It's funny how someone can make you the happiest you could possibly be. It shows how we need people to keep up happy enough to make others happy. Without connections, it is impossible for us to succeed. This relates to my knee because I am going to need my family's support to get through this long journey.

I love the television show *Lost* because it shows how people get second chances in life and how people either take advantage of it or waste it. I don't want to waste my second chance of having a healthy knee. I need this surgery to work, and I am going to do anything it takes to make sure it does. I know the success of this next surgery will have a lot to do with me doing the necessary work. I need to be dedicated to my physical therapy and recovery to make sure my knee is strong and healthy for a lifetime. This is why this show *Lost* means a lot to me because I see myself in a lot of the characters. Second chances are so important. I'm starting to understand that my goal now is to get my knee healthy much more than thinking about getting back on the soccer field. The surgeon said that to me and it didn't sink in until just now.

Recently I have taken up crocheting and I am loving it so far. I find it very therapeutic, and I love to try different things with it. I keep improving and it is slowly showing in my work. Obviously, I have a lot of room for improvement, but I can see myself getting really good at it. Crochet is something that I have been putting my new extra time into and I know I will be sticking with it for a long time.

I've had a lot more downtime to think things over and realized that being kind to a mean person is a strong reflection of your character. It doesn't have as much to do with the other person's character. This means that no matter what another person is doing and how they treat you, you can always do your best to treat them and others with kindness and respect. This shows the type of person that you are. When someone isn't kind to me, I try to think about what the person could be going through and it becomes a little easier for me to be kind to them.

The Women's World Cup is coming up and I am so excited! This is my favorite event ever and I have been waiting for this for such a long time. The men's World Cup was fun, but I enjoy watching women's soccer a bit more. The men tend to flop on the ground way too much. I am so happy because some of my favorite players are on the US women's team, and I can't wait for it to completely consume my life for the next few months. I still love soccer! I just hope that the USA can win! It makes me sad that I will watch soccer realizing that I'm not likely to ever play again. That reality is starting to sink it.

I am really getting into crocheting as a way to occupy my time while I'm preparing for my next surgery. It is very hard for me when I have little else to do, so it is necessary for me to always have a hobby. Right now, I am working on making a tank top and it feels good to be excelling at something.

Staying hydrated is so important for me but sometimes I find myself forgetting to drink water. Funny, I have no issue drinking coffee, but I don't drink nearly enough water. They say that staying hydrated is important for knee health so I'm trying to be better at that. I know that staying hydrated is so crucial for me to have a strong and healthy knee. Starting now, I am going to focus on drinking more water so I can feel good and also have my knee get healthy. I am using a water bottle to help me drink water so I can drink more at one time.

This week, I've been feeling tired. I realize that I sleep in my bed, eat in my bed, watch TV in my bed, etc. I talked to my mom about this, and she told me that I need to force myself to stay away from my bed and only use my bed for sleep. This is going to be really hard for me but maybe if I start doing this, I will have more energy for working on strengthening my knee for my next surgery. I am going to try this out and hopefully see results.

I am trying to think of different ways to get exercise. Since I can't do much as my knee is still very unstable, I need to find new ways to exercise. So far, I am riding the stationary bike for short periods four times a day. I talked to my physical therapist, and he said I can start swimming. I am scared about this as I worry that something could happen, and I could get injured. I hope that I can get past my fears and focus on what is best for my recovery and me. I haven't tried swimming in so long so maybe it would be nice to do it again.

I am getting better and better at crochet as time goes by. Right now, I'm working on a shirt for my sister for which I am very excited. It is very time consuming, but I know that all things that take time are worth it in the end. Another thing that I have been working on is doing more physical therapy at home outside of my sessions with my physical therapist. Doing the work on my own will help me gain strength back in my knee and throughout my whole body.

I have been swimming almost every single day and I can say that it is really helping my knee improve. Ever since I started swimming, I feel like I have had better range of motion with my knee and just feel stronger. It is also good to get in the sun which apparently helps the body produce more vitamin D. I have missed swimming and it's something that I'm going to stick with throughout the summer.

We still haven't decided a date on my surgery. We are going back and forth on which option would be best. My parents want me to push back the surgery closer to

December, but I want to get the surgery done as soon as possible. The Taylor Swift concert is coming up. She's my all-time favorite musician and I really want to go to the concert. That would mean so much to me. I'm nervous about attending the concert in a knee brace after the surgery, but it looks like the next surgery will be after the concert, so it won't be an issue. For the next surgery, they will need to use some of right knee patella tendon to fix the ACL on my "bad" left knee. Since the surgery will affect both of my legs, I'm going to be having to take a lot of rest following my surgery.

Today at physical therapy, I had a moment where my knee started to feel unstable. I haven't had this happen since my second surgery because, so far, my knee has felt pretty stable even though I don't have a complete ACL there. Feeling the instability is really scary for me because it felt close to what it felt like when I tore my ACL and my meniscus. Obviously, my knee is okay, but something just moved a little in my knee, if that makes sense. But, for a second, I thought that I did tear my ACL or my meniscus again. It was really scary for me to go through that because the last thing I need is another incident where I tear something in my knee.

My physical therapist told me that as I progress, I'm going to start noticing the fact that I don't have a complete ACL in my knee anymore. He said that there is going to be a time where I will reach a plateau and will need to just stay at that certain level until I have surgery so that I do not injure my knee. At this point, I am just trying to gain strength back in my knee and get ready for my next surgery. I am not in the recovery process yet, but I still want to get strength back in my knee so that I can go into the surgery with the best situation possible.

I love being at physical therapy now. The environment is so amazing. I love being at physical therapy because everyone is so nice and comforting. It is such a positive environment and I love going to physical therapy. The exercising part can get very difficult but I still love being there, and I look forward to it every day.

Happiness and confidence are the prettiest things you can wear. If you have happiness and confidence in your life, you automatically present yourself nicer. It is all about the way that you demonstrate kindness and happiness in your daily life. It is not as important to wear nice clothes and have expensive jewelry. If you are not beautiful on the inside, then you can never be truly beautiful on the outside. People can see deep down if a person is really happy and confident, and it is always beautiful to see people who show that side of themselves to everyone around them.

If somebody hurts you, it's okay to cry a river. Just remember to build a bridge and get over it. Every single person has a moment in their life where they struggle, and they have a moment of weakness. It is how you respond to that weak spot in your life and how you make yourself better from the situation that determines how you grow as a person. Every situation should help you become stronger. It should allow you to grow as a person and help make those experiences worth it in the long run. Every experience builds character and makes you stronger.

Those who bring sunshine into the lives of others cannot keep it from themselves. If I am unhappy then there is no possibility that I can make other people happy as well. Before I can focus on having good quality friends, I need to treat myself with respect. I often forget that I need to take care of myself rather than just trying to please others around me. Sometimes I forget that I am a person who deserves to be happy. We all are.

For every minute you are angry, you lose sixty seconds of happiness. I tend to forget that my happiness is determined by how I am as a person. Every time I'm angry, that is a moment wasted where I could have lived life to the fullest. I need to stop wasting time by being angry over insignificant things that I can't change. For example, instead of being angry about my knee issues, I can look on the bright side of life. I have so much in life for which to be grateful.

Joy does not simply happen to us. We must choose joy and keep choosing it every day. Being happy is an option, but it can be difficult to do. Happiness takes work and it's something that we must give into the world. Ultimately, this makes us happy as well. It is up to us to have a positive outlook on life and be a kind and genuine person. Therefore, I can't just assume that joy will come to me without putting in the effort.

There's only one happiness in this life; to love and be loved. Happiness is the action of being good to others and hoping that others will be good to you. It is a transaction as it goes both ways. If you want to be happy and to be loved, you have to be loving to others as well. It's not a one-way street where you can just get the good side of life without sharing that with others. I sometimes forget that I have to send out good energy to others if I want to receive back good energy.

MY FAVORITE QUOTES

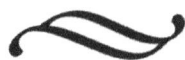

I've been thinking a lot about what makes people happy, and I've been reading a lot of wonderfully inspiring quotes. Music and television shows are very important to me and have been great sources of quotes that have helped me through my ACL recovery.

The TV show Ted Lasso has a bunch of amazing quotes that have stuck with me for many years. The first quote that sticks out to me is "Doing the right thing is never the wrong thing." This quote is special because it shows that something can seem hard but can still be the right thing to do. You can always tell if something is right or wrong based on what result is likely to happen. For example, think about what is likely to happen if you say something to someone in your life. Is the result likely to be good or bad? I mean the long-term result, not the short-term result. Sometimes, we need to say something to someone, and the initial result may not be positive. However, it may still be the right thing to say. This just shows that most things in life have either a good or bad long-term result and doing the right thing is never the wrong thing. The way I think about this is that I think about whether I'm saying something with goodness in my heart or negative feelings in my heart. If I'm saying it with goodness and kindness in my heart, then it's usually the right thing. This relates to my knee as I need to take good care of my knee and do the "right things" that would lead to good circumstances in the future.

Another quote that is very important to me is "I think things come into our lives to help us get from one place to a better one." This is very special to me because there have been many things to happen in my life recently that have helped lead to something better. For instance, if I had never torn my ACL, I would have never discovered crocheting and I would have never met certain friends that I have today. Also, I would not be the strong person I am today. I have grown so much as an individual and have learned so many new things that have helped shape the person I am today. I would still rather not have torn my ACL but do realize that there have been some positives because of the path that put me on.

In addition, there is another quote that is very important to me. It is "Taking on a challenge is a lot like riding a horse, isn't it? If you're comfortable while you're doing it, you're probably doing it wrong." This quote really encapsulates how the recovery process for my ACL has been. If it had been a very smooth and easy process, then I wouldn't have grown nearly as much and probably wouldn't be as far along in my recovery as I am. Furthermore, I know that I can't expect everything to come easily for me. That's not how life is, and I need to know that there has to be challenges in my life in order for me to grow.

The quote "The harder you work, the luckier you get" really shows how you must put in the work in order to be successful in life. If I want to have a healthy knee, I need to put in the hours towards my physical therapy in order for that to happen. I can't just expect to wake up one day with a healthy knee. In order for me to be successful, I need to put in the time in order for that to come true. No one is just "lucky" that things turn out well for them, it takes hard work to get a positive result. Success comes from time and what you do with that time. And, if I work hard, I am likely to have a better result (get lucky) than if I don't.

The quote from Ted Lasso "You say impossible, but all I hear is 'I'm possible'" is very interesting if you think about it. It is a play on words saying that the word impossible can also be turned into the sentence "I'm possible." This just comes to show that nothing in life is impossible, and anything can happen if you put in the amount of effort it takes to make that happen. I can't just look at something and say, "Oh that's impossible I could never do that," without actually trying first. There have been many times where I have almost given up on trying to make my knee strong and healthy again. I just need to remember that success takes time and effort and believing that you can succeed.

Another quote that is very significant to me is "It's not the years in your life that count, but rather the life in your years." This quote is very interesting to think about because it's talking about how there has to be many significant moments in your life that can change the way that you live. And it points out that what is important is not just the months and years passing but what you do during that time. Throughout the last year there have been many moments that changed the way that I am as a person. My life has gone through many different things. I have gone through many different stages in my life, and I've realized that it's what I went through in those years that have made me the person I am today. The "life" in those years made me stronger. I tore my ACL. I made new friends. I lost friends. I went through so many different things in my life that changed the way that I live. Looking back, I can't believe how much life there was in those years.

The quote "Life is 10%, what happens to you and 90% how you respond to it," relates a lot to what I'm going through right now and what I've been through. My ACL tear was just one small moment in my life, but the way that I responded to that significant event has been far more important. I have gone through over a year of physical therapy and have had two surgeries and will need to have another soon. There have been many moments where I wanted to stop doing physical therapy because I felt weak along this journey. However, I kept going. It was the way that I responded to that significant event that was far more important than the event in question.

"The greatest day in life is when we take total responsibility for our attitudes. That's the day we truly grow up." This quote by John C. Maxwell truly encapsulates the journey that I have been travelling for the last year and am still on today. I had spent much time not fully accepting my responsibility in this process. The second that I finally looked in the mirror and realized that my recovery is up to me is when I grew as a person.

The quote from Ted Lasso "Just listen to your gut, and on the way down to your gut, check in with your heart and they'll let you know what's what," genuinely describes how I've been making decisions. I realize that I have to listen to my gut, but I also have to follow my heart. There is a fine line between doing what you feel is right and what I know is right. I have to listen to both my gut and my heart to make the right decisions. It may not feel right at the moment, but if your gut is telling you that it's right and your heart is telling you that's right, then there's almost 100% certainty that that is the right thing to do.

When I'm struggling about my knee surgery and my recovery, I think about the quote "It may not work out how you think it will or how you hope it does, but believe me, it will all work out." I know that not everything in life will go 100% the way I want it to go, but it eventually will work itself out. I have to go with the flow sometimes and realize that I might just have to live with the fact that I may never play soccer again. However, this could be a blessing in disguise. Maybe I will learn new things and discover new hobbies that I would have never discovered if I had been able to stay with soccer.

Here is the new quote of the day; "Do what is right, not what is easy." There are many things in life that might seem to be the easier options. However, they might not be the right things to do. You know deep down what is the right thing to do. Sometimes the right thing to do is the harder option. I struggle with coming to terms with this, because I tend to gravitate towards the easier option rather than the right option. This has caused me to limit myself to possibilities and limit myself to what I am capable of being. This won't be the case going forward. Doing the right thing comes before doing the easy thing.

"It takes time to create excellence. If it could be done quickly, more people would do it." I think about this often when I think about all of my goals in life. I now want to be a sports broadcaster and journalist so, obviously, I know that's going to take a lot of work. I mean, it would be convenient if the desirable thing in life was the easy thing to do, but obviously, that is not the case. If everything in life came easy, then there would be no motivation to work hard at anything. What motivates us is the challenges that we must overcome. That makes us stronger and, ultimately, happier people.

"Failing to prepare is preparing to fail." Preparation is so important. It is almost like setting yourself up for failure if you do not go into a situation with full preparation. There is almost no situation or job in life which requires no preparation. Everything in life must come with care and preparation so that you can do a quality job. I need to remember that I can't just live my life hoping that I can force greatness without actually working hard to get there. As the saying goes, Rome wasn't built in a day. I can't just wake up one day and assume that all of my problems will be solved. None of my goals will be achieved without the hard work that it takes to get there.

"Don't let yesterday take up too much of today." This is very meaningful to me because it reminds me that I can't let what happened in the past prevent me from living in the present. I can't just go about living every day thinking about what I should have done or what I wish didn't happen in the past. I need to worry about the future as well as the present in order to live a full life. As the saying goes from Ted Lasso, "Goldfish are the happiest animals because their memory only lasts five seconds." Goldfish are able to live in the moment, because they forget about what just happened five seconds prior. I should start living like a goldfish and live every moment to the fullest and not focus on what happened the previous day.

"Listen if you want to be heard." I know that respect is a two-way street and yet I sometimes expect people to treat me a certain way without treating them that same way. We learned when we were little the Golden Rule which is to treat others the way we want to be treated. I need to remember that people will treat me the same way that I treat them. I need to focus on treating every single person I come across with the utmost respect in order for me to expect that they will treat me with that same respect.

The song "Never Grow Up" by Taylor Swift is really important to me because the lyrics talk about all the universal experiences that a person goes through growing up. For example, when people are young, they always want to feel older and have more responsibilities, but as soon as you get closer to adulthood, you find yourself wishing that you had appreciated your youth more. I am going through that right now as I turn 18 in less than 2 months.

"Rise above the storm and you will find the sunshine." This quote summarizes how I am struggling with looking on the bright side and finding the good in my situation. When I think about my future surgery, all I focus on is the negatives. I need to think positively and realize that after this surgery, I can finally have a healthy knee. Instead of worrying about the bad, I need to look for the good, as that is a better way to look at life. If I do this, it will be so much easier to find happiness. There is sunshine just about the storm and I'm starting to see a break in the clouds.

"Be the change you wish to see in the world." If I want things to change in the world, I need to be proactive and make changes happen in my own life. I can't just assume that things will change as long as I stay the way I am. If I want to have a strong knee, I have to make that happen with my own actions. I can't just wish for it to happen without putting in the hours of work it takes for that to happen.

"The only person you are destined to become is the person you decide to be." I like to assume I am a certain way, but at the same time, my actions need to always reflect that. If I want to be a good person, I need to always act in kind and compassionate ways both to others and to myself. I can't pretend to be good. It must be real and authentic.

"If you want the rainbow, you gotta put up with the rain." Nothing good and real ever comes easy. Life takes effort. I know that I have to struggle and do a lot of painful physical therapy in order to get the end result of having a normal and strong knee. This takes time, but all good things come with time and dedication. I just have to think about what I am working towards and know that all of this is worth it in the end.

"You never really learn much from hearing yourself speak." I have to stop thinking that I know everything and that I know all the answers to my problems. This is a foolish way to live, and I need to get better at asking for help. This starts with listening a lot more. We have two ears and one mouth so I guess we should do twice as much listening as talking. And the more I listen, the more I learn, which is always a good thing. And, if I can just take in the love people are showing me, I will be much happier.

"Life isn't how to survive the storm; it's about how to dance in the rain." This quote demonstrates how it is all how you handle a situation, and how you find the good in every situation. If you only look for the negative, you will never have the ability to be able to see everything good that is right in front of you. Every single situation has a silver lining, but it is up to us to find it.

"I'd rather regret what didn't work out than the chances I didn't take it all." There have been many moments where I was too scared to take a risk and then I regretted that decision later on. I need to stop living my life like that, because it keeps me from trying things that I might be successful at. I would much rather regret something not working out than regretting not trying at all. I believe this is a much better way to live.

"One person practicing sportsmanship is far better than fifty preaching it." I think about this quote quite a bit. Actions speak louder than words. Doing something is far better than just talking about it. If you believe in something, take action. Be the leader who takes action. I'm speaking from personal experience when I say that it is not as important to say that you're going to do something instead of actually doing it.

"A trophy carries dust. Memories last forever." A trophy might seem nice, but the memories that you made while earning the trophy are far more important. I think about every time my team won a soccer trophy and all I can remember is the memories from that day. I can look up at my trophy stand and see all of them sitting there. However, what I really remember is the happiness and joy that I felt when I won each of them. That is the true meaning behind the trophies.

"Set your goals high, and don't stop until you get there." It is always important to have high standards for yourself and you should set goals for yourself that push you to be better. If you just stay at the same level that you are right now, you will never improve in life. If I just set easy and quick goals for myself, then I will obviously succeed, but I will never improve as a person. This will just limit me and make it so I will never truly be great.

Set high standards for yourself, but also remember to keep working until you reach your goals.

"The difference between the impossible and the possible lies in a man's determination." We are taught from a very young age that nothing is impossible, and everything is possible. However, we aren't always taught the secret to make things possible. I've learned that it's called grit. Grit is a combination of determination, patience, and perseverance.

"Show me someone who's afraid to look bad, and I'll show you someone you can beat in soccer every time." That goes for just about any activity. Our focus shouldn't be on how we look, but rather how we're doing. Are we improving? Are we learning new skills? Fearing what others think limits us and holds us back. For example, there were times playing soccer where I was afraid of looking bad, so I didn't make that risky play and it limited me from scoring more goals. I'm now working hard to focus on how I'm doing in life, rather than worrying about what others think as that will ultimately make me happier as well as more successful.

Sportsmanship for me is when someone walks off the court and you really can't tell whether he or she has won or lost. These sorts of people carry themselves with pride either way. They focus on the performance and being in the moment rather than the result. I've heard coaches call this focusing on the process rather than the result. In this sense, excellence is not a singular act, but a group of habits practiced in a consistent manner. We are what we do repeatedly. It's more important to do the correct things over and over again instead of focusing on a given result. Greatness is when we normalize performing at an elite level, when we have the process down to a science over and over again. Focusing on process over results is also found in the quote "It's not the will to win that matters, it's the will to prepare to win that matters." Following the right process is the key.

"No matter what happens in life, be good to people. Being good to people is a wonderful legacy to leave behind." This is such an important quote and concept. There is nothing more important than being kind to others; especially those who are vulnerable. You learn a lot about a person's character based on how they treat other people, especially people they perceive as having a lower status. Being good to people reveals our true character.

My Philosophy

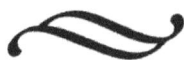

I've had a lot of time to think and reflect on my philosophy of life since I first tore my ACL. This has helped me come to some realizations that now shape my worldview and how I approach my life and the people in it. I would give anything to have never torn my ACL, but I do think my new perspective is a blessing.

No matter how bad your day is, just be grateful this day is added to your life. Every day is a blessing. It may be a cliché, but it is a blessing just to be alive. Every day is a blessing, and I am so fortunate to be able to wake up and have good health and be able to enjoy each moment. Even though difficult things may happen, it is still a blessing that we have this day. It's a gift and I need to remember to always treat it like one. We should always treat it that way. I hope that you have received some benefit from my experience without, I hope, having to go through the same situation.

AVIGAIL'S TOP TEN LISTS

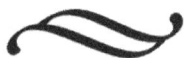

Top Questions To Ask Your Surgeon

1. How many ACL surgeries do you perform each month?

2. Do you have a physical therapy program for your patients to follow after surgery?

3. Do you have any recommended physical therapists?

4. Which ACL grafts do you use for your surgeries and why?

5. What are the pros and cons of each graft?

6. How do you determine when a patient can get back on the field?

7. What percentage of your patients get back on the field within 12 months?

Top Questions To Ask Your Physical Therapist

1. How many ACL patients do you take care of each month?

2. How do you provide feedback to the surgeons?

3. With which surgeons do you see the best results?

4. Which grafts do you find have the best results?

5. What percentage of your patients get back on the field within 12 months?

Top Stress Reducers During Your Recovery

1. Meditation

2. Siting with a dog or cat

3. Spending time in nature, especially near a mountain or water if that's possible

4. Listening to music

5. Reading a book

6. Hanging out with friends

Top Ten Secrets For Better Sleep

1. Wake up and go to bed at about the same time every day (even on weekends)

2. Don't eat or drink three hours before bedtime

3. No caffeine after noon

4. Don't do anything super stressful after 6 p.m. (no news or scary movies)

5. Avoid smartphones, tablets, or computers an hour before bedtime.

6. Don't exercise within four hours of bedtime

7. Use lavender essential oils to scent your room

8. Don't nap during the day (if you do, nothing over 30 minutes)

Top Nutrition Tips Before and After Surgery (please review with your doctor)

1. Focus on non-processed foods meaning there are five or fewer ingredients on the label

2. Avoid highly processed carbohydrates

3. Make sure you get enough protein

4. Hydrate

5. Don't eat within three hours of bedtime

CONCLUSION

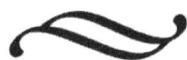

Here we are at the end of the book. It may be the end of the book, but it's not the end of my, or your, journey. The main lesson I've learned on my ACL journey is that our journeys never truly end. We continue them as long as we walk the Earth and then we pass on our journeys to the next generation. I've learned that we don't really have separate journeys, but rather we travel our journeys alongside each other. Your journey impacts those close to you and so on. Sorry to wax a bit poetic here, when we look at things like this, we realize that part of life is about taking one step at a time and moving forward, rather than backward. Looking back on what's happened, both the good and the bad, is a common thing to do, but it's rarely productive. Doing so tends to pull us into the abyss of negative patterns. Instead, I try to focus less on what could have been and more on what could be next. My goal is to bring where I've been and what I've experienced into the present moment to make today a beautiful gem.

For me, playing soccer was something I loved, and I treasured every darn moment of it. However, that's now a part of my past and the only question that I face today is what I can take from that experience and live in this current moment. My focus is on how I can create more wonderful moments. As Billy Joel once said, "I'm warm from the memory of days to come." How can we stay warm as we create new memories each day? That's what I've learned on my ACL Journey. I've learned that life is a journey of rediscovering or rebooting ourselves each day, both with the memories of our past and the hope of the days yet to come. Where does your journey take you next? Where does my journey take me next? I love soccer. I love sports. I really do. I love the drama. I love the discipline and the preparation that goes into getting ready for games. I love the games themselves where we learn who we are and what we're made of deep inside.

I love everything about sports, and I've realized that I have a passion and a joy sharing all this with others. This book is one way that I've expressed this love and sports broadcasting, and journalism is another. I've been taking broadcasting courses at my high school for the last four years and I love it so much. Playing soccer may not be in the cards for me going forwards, but sharing my love of sports with others sure can be. I can help others see the beauty of sports through broadcasting and journalism. I never would have realized this had it not been for my ordeal. This journey has allowed me to step back from sports and see the wonder of it all and how truly miraculous and life-changing it can be and now I can spend the rest of my journey sharing this joy with others. For me, I'm not sure there is anything more wonderful.

So, this is where I am today on my journey. I've realized that I'm actually just getting started on my life journey as the journey never ends. Life continues to happen and move forward. We're always facing challenges as we move through life. We don't always choose our challenges, but we do have the choice on how we respond to these changes. How do we see these events? Do we see them as catastrophes or as challenges to grow and discover more about ourselves? I've learned that is the true struggle of life; the struggle to see our "pops" as opportunities rather than catastrophes. I've talked so much here about me, but it's not just about me. This is about all of us because we're all on a journey. In some ways, each of our journeys is separate and distinct, but in another sense, our journeys share so much in common. I sincerely hope that some of my experiences have helped you on your path. The details of our journeys may be different, but the lessons are the same. Right now, I don't know what is going to happen, but I am optimistic it's going to be amazing. I will keep you posted.

Avigail

ACKNOWLEDGEMENTS

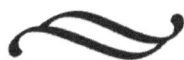

Thank you, Mom and Dad. Thank you so much for being my role models for how to live a life of happiness, meaning, and service to others. I am so grateful to both of you for teaching me to never give up on myself. I love you.

I also want to thank Camp Kesem for providing me with lasting and meaningful friendships that supported me during the difficult times as my mom battled cancer. My Kesem friends have given me the best summer weeks and helped me through so many landmarks in my life. Camp Kesem is working towards a world where no child has to deal with a parent's cancer alone and I fully support them and their life-changing mission.

Information About The Author

Avigail Morris is a senior at a high school just outside Los Angeles, CA. Avigail began playing soccer at age three and club soccer at age six. Avigail played on an Elite Club National League soccer team for many years with the Camarillo Eagles Soccer Club. She was the season MVP for her high school varsity soccer team. She is now continuing her journey off the soccer pitch, planning on a career in sports journalism. Avigail is the third of four children.

www.ingramcontent.com/pod-product-compliance
Lightning Source LLC
Chambersburg PA
CBHW021336290326
41933CB00038B/824